WORKING

on the

Ball

WORKING

on the

Ball

A **Simple Guide** *to* **Office Fitness**

Jane Clapp

Sarah Robichaud

Andrews McMeel
Publishing

Kansas City

06 07 08 09 10 TWP 10 9 8 7 6 5 4 3 2 1

ISBN-13: 978-0-7407-5699-3
ISBN-10: 0-7407-5699-0

Library of Congress Control Number: 2005052961

www.andrewsmcmeel.com

Photography by Michael Alberstat
www.alberstat.com

Design by Pete Lippincott

Contents

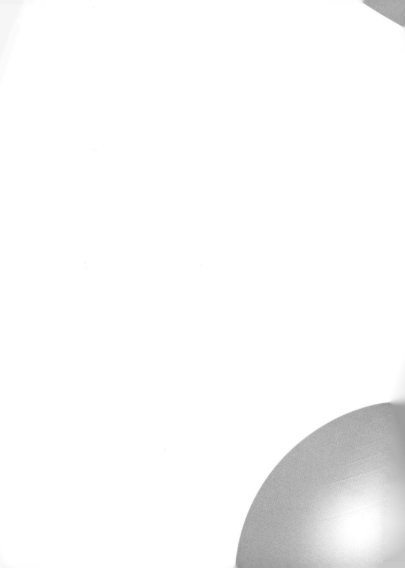

Getting on the Ball

Working on the Ball in a Nutshell

Working on the Ball throws the acclaimed fitness tool into a new arena: *the workplace,* where most of us spend most of our time. We provide an innovative and playful approach to fitness—no gym shoes or expensive fitness club memberships required. We don't use lots of fitness jargon and we don't expect you to take yourself too seriously. We want to help you find the strong, sexy, and powerful you. If you do what we tell you to do, you will.

We take you through a full day of exercises to be performed at your desk while using a stability ball as a chair (also referred to as "active sitting"). We share useful tips for immediate lifestyle improvements to help you make healthy choices at work. And we're there with you, on each page, to coach, to demonstrate, and to cheer you on.

Do You *Sit at a Computer* Most of the Day?

Anyone can deduce that sitting and slouching at a desk all day is hazardous to lower-back health and posture. In addition to making the worst of our nine-to-five activity, it can lead to such physical conditions as kyphosis (rounding of the upper back and shoulders) and lordosis (excessive curvature in the lower back). These conditions contribute to neck pain, headaches, dull lower-back pain, decreased enjoyment of life, and an unattractive appearance. Headaches and lower-back pain (in that order) are the most frequent pain ailments, according to the Mayo Clinic in Rochester, Minnesota. A full 70 percent of the population experiences lower-back pain every year. Even though people blame their workplaces for lower-back pain and all kinds of other ailments, they remain out of touch with what their bodies really need: to eat less and move more.

These conditions are just as bad for business as they are for employees. Work-related back injuries are the most common type of injury, involving the most lost workdays. The trunk, including the shoulder and back, is the body part most affected by work incidents, accounting for 36.5 percent of all 2001 claims (U.S. Bureau of Labor Statistics, 2003).

Meanwhile, growing awareness of the importance of more mindful living has created a huge market for preventative health care, as well as for exercise that is more accessible.

Roughly seventy million Americans use a computer. There's something mesmerizing about computers. We can sit in the same posture for an hour or two and forget about the passage of time. Computers have changed the nature of our economy and the nature of the way we use our bodies.

You think working on a construction site is dangerous? Working at a computer isn't as safe as you might like to believe. Sitting and slouching at your desk all day will make your job hazardous to good posture and back health.

There are many different possible causes for bad posture, but the most likely is a lack of awareness when sitting at your desk, the place where you spend potentially 40 to 50 percent of your waking hours. You might even be on your way to developing kyphosis or lordosis. In addition, sitting still and not moving all day can lead to excess fat storage and a big flabby butt.

We are a knowledge and information society. Knowledge workers think for a living. But your thinking becomes impaired when you stop moving for prolonged periods. The great news is that being active and working on the ball will pay off not only for your body but for your work as well. If you can keep your body in motion, you can keep your mind in motion.

Working on the Ball Tackles the North American *Health Crisis*

What we're going to talk about isn't pretty. If you're not convinced that you need to address your own health and fitness now, this section is *very* important for you. Even though people are spending more money on gym memberships, fitness books, and exercise equipment, North Americans are getting fatter and fatter. Obesity trends for the United States show a dramatic increase year after year. In 1991, four states reported obesity prevalence rates of 15 to 19 percent and no states reported a rate above 20 percent. In 2002, eighteen states had obesity rates of 15 to 19 percent: Twenty-nine states had rates of 20 to 24 percent and three states had rates over 25 percent. Right now, 64 percent of Americans are overweight or obese. Health complications from obesity and inactivity will soon be the number-one cause of early mortality in America. Clearly, something isn't working.

One of the main reasons for these increases is the environment in which people spend many of their waking hours: work. Work environments provide barriers to opportunity for an active lifestyle (Centers for Disease Control and Prevention, 2002). According to the National Institute for Occupational Safety and Health, seventy million workers in the United States use a computer. The majority of them are in front of the keyboard all day. When they're not at work, they may be sitting in a car or on a bus or train. Commuters now spend 14 percent more time commuting than they did in 1990, an average increase of more than thirty minutes per day (U.S. Department of Labor, 2003).

The average American spends 1,821 hours working each year. The minimum amount of exercise recommended is 183 hours yearly, or about three and a half hours per week. Fewer than 33 percent of adults engage in the recommended amount of physical activity. And 40 percent of Americans do not participate in any physical activity at all ("Surgeon General's Call to Action to Prevent and Decrease Overweight and Obesity," 2004). Everyone knows they should be physically active on a regular basis, but many say that lack of time is the major impediment. As fitness trainers with corporate experience, we knew what to do. We did a little math. Incorporating those 183 hours into the 1,821 gives people one of the things they most lack. Extra time!

We created *Working on the Ball* to address this major health crisis in North America, which has come about as a result of working conditions and the general lack of discipline regarding healthy living. *Working on the Ball* reaches people in the environment they frequent most: the workplace. It provides a means to exercise while doing what we do anyway: sitting. And it removes some of the barriers to health by making exercise and even work more fun.

A 2004 study in the *Journal of Occupational and Environmental Medicine* found that physically active people were more likely to enjoy their jobs. They also produced higher-quality work and received more positive recognition from their managers. Get ready. Work is about to become a lot more efficient and lucrative!

Many unconditioned people and those who find it difficult to maintain a consistent exercise regimen actually crave engaging and result-focused physical activity. Lots of people find convenient excuses to avoid all exercise because they fear it takes too much time to get fit. People also want to find ways to be active without sacrificing time for other pleasurable activities. In addition, people want to get fit in the shortest time possible, with the least imposition on their lives. Within your eight-hour day, you can get your workout out of the way.

The Cure for **Poor Posture!** *Use a Stability Ball* **as Your Chair**

Having developed poor posture over a lifetime, you'll need restorative muscle building to help you get rid of bad habits. This is where the stability ball comes in. "Functional training" is one of the most-used buzz phrases in fitness today. Functional training's goal is to build strength for day-to-day movements by mimicking how the body is used in real life. This is why most personal trainers and physiotherapists incorporate functional training into their clients' programs. The ball is recognized as an integral tool for functional training. It helps prevent and treat lower-back injury by improving core strength, balance, and coordination. How? The stability ball is *unstable*. And having an unstable surface to sit on automatically activates core muscles in your midsection to keep you balanced. As a result, many fitness professionals recommend using the ball as a chair as a way to change posture and movement patterns and to incorporate core strengthening into busy lives.

If you think about evolution and how the arrangement of human organs housed in a structure of bone and muscle evolved over hundreds of thousands of years, it's easy to see how important balanced sitting is. Until our cushy, comfy modern times, humans were upright and active and relied on strong muscles to maintain an upright sitting position. Relatively recently, desk jobs and padded chairs have turned our posture to mush.

Without a doubt, *active sitting*—a.k.a. using the ball as a chair—improves core strength and posture and keeps our minds more focused on the tasks at hand. Using it, you will reassign responsibility for stability to the muscles that are designed to keep this system in balance. You'll get stronger without even thinking about it. Seem too good to be true? As soon as you sit on a ball, lots of tiny muscles start working. Sit on a ball and try letting your body go limp. *Oops!* Did you fall right off the ball?

Good Posture Is Better Two Ways

Good posture is the absolute foundation of any fitness program, and it will be the key to your success. Since we help people with fitness every day, we know how hard it is to tackle poor posture and to keep it from sneaking back up on you. We also know from working one-on-one with so many clients that the effects of improved posture are immeasurable. So please trust us for now. Improved

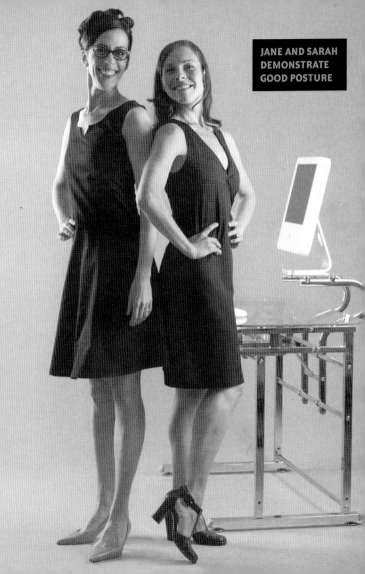

JANE AND SARAH
DEMONSTRATE
GOOD POSTURE

posture is well worth your mental and physical effort. Good posture makes you look confident and strong. And that's not all: It actually *creates* confidence and strength by optimizing the way you feel.

If you think about it, posture communicates a whole "state of being" to the outside world. Look carefully at people with great posture. Their body language says, "I *rock,* I'm ready for anything—bring it on, baby." Their open chest makes them taller and more approachable. They appear more alert and more confident. Now take a close look at people who slouch. Their body language announces, "I've got the blahs. Don't ask me to do anything else. I'm tired and burned out." As an added turnoff, their rounded shoulders make them shorter and closed off, making them appear harder to approach.

The physical benefits of good posture become apparent when you investigate the spine. Note that it consists of the bones (vertebrae) and discs that support the body and protect the spinal cord. There are three curves in the spine: at the neck, midback, and lower back. When these curves are in place, as shown on the next page, it's called the "neutral position."

If one of these curves moves out of alignment, poor posture results, quickly followed by stress and strain on

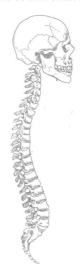

joints and ligaments. The muscles attached to the bones are affected because they can't work efficiently and get tired much faster. Consequently, back and neck muscles get weaker, leading to pain and extra wear and tear.

So the next time you're sitting at your desk, take time to analyze how you're holding your body. Begin with your head. Is it jutting forward? The more tired you get, the more your head will stick out over your neck. Did you know that

ABNORMAL, UNHAPPY SPINAL CURVATURE

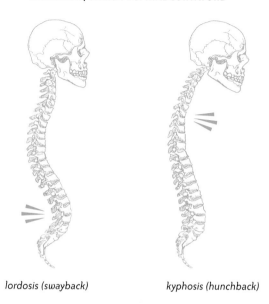

lordosis (swayback)   *kyphosis (hunchback)*

the average human head weighs eight to twelve pounds?
For every inch your head moves forward, your neck muscles
assume an extra fifteen to thirty pounds of weight. This
automatically throws off your posture, and your body begins
to compensate for the shift. Your shoulders become rounded,
and a hump begins to develop in your upper back. The

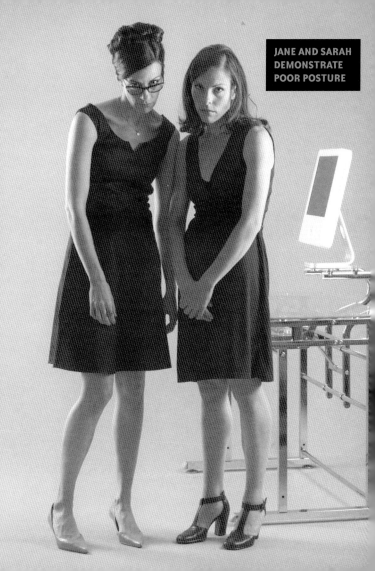

JANE AND SARAH
DEMONSTRATE
POOR POSTURE

results can be neck and back pain, tension, and even headaches. No wonder deskwork feels like a pain in the neck!

Poor posture also precipitates physical stress by restricting the optimum physiological processes of your lungs and other organs. When a drooping torso inhibits or irritates the nerves coming out of your spine or keeps your rib cage from expanding and contracting, it stresses and puts pressure on organs and tissues in the chest and lower torso.

Generalized lower-back pain is quite common, and is usually treatable. The combination therapy is losing weight (if necessary), increasing joint flexibility, improving core strength, and improving posture. Working on the ball can provide all of these outcomes. Nevertheless, we don't want to trivialize severe lower-back pain, because it can point to a bigger problem.

Call your doctor immediately if:

- You have any concerns about undiagnosed pain anywhere in your back or neck.

- You feel numbness, tingling, or loss of control in your arms or legs.

- The pain in your back extends downward along the back of your leg.

- The pain increases when you cough or bend forward at the waist.

- The pain is accompanied by fever.

- You have dull pain in one area of your spine when lying in or getting out of bed.

Checking *Your Own Posture*

A good way to figure out whether you have a slumping problem is to assess your own posture. Here's an easy way to see how you hold yourself. As you begin applying the techniques in this book to work on your physique, use this method to check how much you're improving your posture.

- Stand with your heels against a wall, knees slightly bent.

- Your palms should face your thighs and your thumbs should face forward.

- Your calves, butt, back of your shoulders, and back of your head should also touch the wall without you having to tilt your head back or lift your chin up.

- You should be able to slip your hand behind the small of your back.

- Step away from the wall and stand normally.

- Determine what part of your body shifted when you stepped away.

- Correct your posture immediately.

Anytime you feel like you can't get a handle on good posture, put your back up against the wall and help your body remember.

Remember that cautionary adage "Don't make that terrible face because it might stay that way"? Well, the same advice goes for your spine, muscles, organs, eyes, and body in general. Consider whether you stand and sit straight or whether you're more inclined to slump like a sack of potatoes in your chair. If you sit all day with poor posture and relaxed stomach muscles, your body remembers and maintains the look of a misshapen gunnysack even when you're not at your desk. No one wants to look this way and no one wants the health problems that may result.

Choosing a Ball

One of the benefits of using a ball as a chair is cost. An ergonomically correct chair often costs $500 and up, whereas an excellent-quality stability ball costs only around

$30. For that amount, you might even get your employer to spring for it. You never know until you ask.

Balls are available in a range of prices and levels of quality. Use your judgment about what texture of ball is best for you. The shinier the ball, and the more transparent, usually the less durable. The more rubbery the ball, usually the tougher and more comfortable. Remember that you'll be putting your butt on this ball for what may be all day long. Comfort is an important factor in making your workday the best it can be.

Here are some guidelines for matching height to ball size:

Under 4'8"	45-centimeter (17-inch) ball
4'8"–5'3"	55-centimeter (21-inch) ball
5'4"–6'0"	65-centimeter (25-inch) ball
6'1"–6'7"	75-centimeter (29-inch) ball

These are general guidelines. You still need to try out the ball to make sure it accommodates your leg length.

When you're sitting on the ball, your hips should be at a ninety-degree or slightly larger angle to your legs. If your height is right between the specifications, you may need the larger size if you have long legs or carry extra weight for your

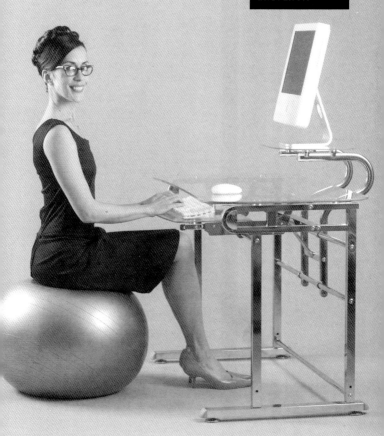

JANE
DEMONSTRATING
PROPER FIT

height. If in doubt, buy a larger ball because it can be slightly underinflated. Usually, you can inflate or deflate the ball to make it fit better. The softer the ball, the less challenging the exercises and active sitting will be, because more surface area touches the ground. The firmer the ball, the more difficult. Follow the manufacturer's guidelines when it comes to filling your ball with air.

Stability-Ball Safety

Use common sense. Don't sit next to a heating vent or anything else hot. Don't sit on top of the broken glass from the martini soirée last night. Don't sit near stairs, open landings, and the like. And, if you have any injury or chronic illness or if you're pregnant, discuss using the ball as a chair with your doctor. In general, you should consult your doctor before starting any new exercise program.

Avoiding Eyestrain *and* Brain Drain

In addition to all the postural issues already discussed, your eyes may suffer from your hours spent hunched over a computer screen. Computer vision syndrome (CVS) encompasses a variety of vision-related problems that can be caused or aggravated by regular computer use (two or more hours per day). Symptoms of CVS can include eye fatigue, dry and burning eyes, headaches, and pain in your neck, shoulders, and back.

Here's how the problem starts. When you stare at a computer screen, your blink rate decreases by 66 percent. Your eyes also get tired from the reflections on your monitor. You may look for a way to sit to avoid the glare. The more strained your eyes get, the more tension you hold in your head and neck muscles. As you can imagine, CVS contributes to whatever effects you suffer from poor posture. To avoid CVS you need to:

- Take a break every twenty minutes by looking away from your computer screen and focusing on another object. The exercises in this book will help you do this.

- Perform the neck and upper-back stretches in this book several times a day.

- Continually realign your posture.

- Remember to blink!

Quick Tips *for Desk Setup*

The affordable ball automatically helps create an ergonomically correct workstation for less. Analyze your current desk setup to see what other modifications are possible. Here are some tips to help prevent your desk setup from interfering with the progress that *Working on the Ball* will provide:

- The top of your computer screen should be at eye level or 20 or 30 degrees below. If you wear bifocals, position your screen low enough so you don't have to tilt your head back to see it. If this isn't possible, given the nonadjustable height of your stability ball, think about getting an adjustable-height computer desk. You can find desks that aren't particularly costly.

- Place the keyboard close to your body, so your elbows are at your sides and bent at a ninety-degree angle.

- Keep the keyboard and mouse on the same level.
- Make sure you don't have to extend your arm to use the mouse.
- Try to keep your wrists in a flat, neutral position over the keyboard.
- To reduce glare, position your screen at a right angle to the window.

Some changes are better than none. Don't get caught in the trap of all-or-nothing thinking. Making even some of the changes listed above will help you in the long run.

Treat Active Sitting as an Endurance Sport

Don't throw away your office chair yet. Sitting on the ball is an endurance activity. You might have to work your way up to being able to use it for a full workday. If you haven't been regularly active for three months or more and haven't been doing any core strengthening, try switching between your regular office chair and the ball. Start using the ball for five to ten minutes every hour until your core gets stronger. Listen to your body and don't expect big changes in your endurance right away. Add more time per hour each week, and before you know it you'll be a complete convert. You'll be preaching the gospel of *Working on the Ball*, you trendsetter you!

It All *Adds Up*

Working on the Ball helps you exercise in short snippets without interrupting your day. If you're committed to being fit, strong, and healthy, accept that you have to work at it every day. Unlike office work, there are no off days. Choices you make minute by minute, hour by hour, day by day add up to either a healthy lifestyle or an unhealthy one.

- Taking the stairs, walking to work—things you can do for a few minutes throughout your day make a difference.

- You reap the same benefit from thirty minutes of exercise split up into smaller chunks as you would if you did it all at once. There really are no excuses.

- You must think about what you eat and how much you move every day and determine whether you want to be an active healthy person or an inactive over-weight person.

- Mindful living means taking responsibility for the moment-to-moment choices you make. Switch off the autopilot!

Your health and fitness depend on your ability to motivate yourself every day. *Working on the Ball* is here to hold your hand. Don't worry!

Results Experienced
Working on the Ball

After two to three weeks, four to five times per week, of consistently completing most of the exercises and stretches in this book and following the Fit Bytes, you will start to notice improved balance, coordination, core strength and posture. We promise.

After two to three months of consistency and following the Fit Bytes, you will likely relieve lower-back pain, upper-back or neck pain, and feel taller. Your clothes will fit better and you'll experience an increased energy level and ability to focus throughout the day. You will be well on your way to the "I *rock*" state of being.

When you reach this point, you can increase the intensity of the exercises. Check the back of this book for tips on how to do that. Soon you will be ready for *Working on the Ball II: The Advanced Edition*!

Choosing When to Start

*H*ow about right now! Choosing the right time to tackle a lifestyle change is one of the most important factors in determining whether you will be successful in maintaining the change. Still, if your life is currently very stressful, it's important to be cautious and avoid setting the bar too high for yourself. As a realistic way of building exercise into your busy workday, use *Working on the Ball* a few minutes per day for the first week, ten minutes per day the next week, and so on. Don't let the repetition in your work environment take the fun out of working on the ball. Your mind and body will thank you. Be patient with yourself and trust that you will feel and see results.

Begin *with Confidence*

If you start a new endeavor with the belief that you aren't coordinated, you won't be. If you feel low-energy and think you're going to have a crummy day, you will. If you think you aren't going to see results, you won't try as hard as you could. If you think you will never be good at a physical activity, for sure you won't be. And if you believe you are always going to be unhappy with the way you look, you will accept this as an absolute truth. You construct your world and your beliefs. Wishes, positive or negative, do come true.

In contrast, if you start a new endeavor with the belief that you are going to be successful, chances are you will be. If you think you can be coordinated, you will be. If you feel that high energy is achievable and believe you can achieve it, you will. If you are committed to seeing results, you will try as hard as you can. If you aim to excel at a physical activity, you will. And if you believe you are able to be happy with the way you look, you will accept this as an absolute truth. Again, you construct your world and your beliefs. Wishes, positive or negative, do come true.

Working on the Ball and Eating at Your Desk

W hen it comes to what you eat, we don't pretend to have simple answers to an often complicated issue. We do, however, have some ideas that might help you build a healthier desk lifestyle.

Here's the issue: Sitting at your desk might have become an eating trigger for you. You might be eating out of boredom, when you need a pick-me-up, or for emotional reasons, such as after someone has really ticked you off. Do you snack or eat lunch at your desk? Have candies on your desk? Drink coffee at your desk? If so, here are some strategies to use when all you want to do is run to Starbucks and get a big sugary latte and a yummy football-sized pastry.

First, try opening this book to the part of Chapter 2 that corresponds to the time of day you're in. Do some of the exercises. If you're feeling tense, relax by doing some stretches from Chapter 3. Then see if it was just boredom that triggered your desire to eat. If you're still hungry, drink some water. If you're *still* hungry, munch some of the healthy goods listed here.

Stuff you can keep in your drawer for weeks:

- Protein or energy bars
- Trail mix
- Fruit leather with a handful of almonds
- Nut or seed bars
- Dehydrated soups (preferably lentil or bean)
- Sunflower seeds and dried cranberries
- Less processed health-food-store snacks

Stuff for the fridge:

- Precut veggies with a couple of slices of lean deli meat
- Lower-fat yogurt
- Reduced-fat cheese with rye crisps
- Protein and fruit shakes (keep frozen berries in case you run out of fruit)
- Low-fat cottage cheese with fruit and/or sunflower seeds
- Bean or lentil salad
- Lettuce-leaf wrap with tuna inside
- Hard-boiled egg with some veggies or a piece of fruit
- Natural peanut butter or almond butter and rye crisps

Managing Stress *and*
Working on the Ball

It's easy to lose perspective when we get stressed out. Pressure getting to you? No time for everything you need to get done and deadlines piling up? Sometimes the best thing to do is take a break from your computer screen to get out of your head and into your body. Physical activity is one of the best ways to help your brain function optimally. Your work will still be there after your short break, and your mind will be more centered to tackle the task at hand.

If you need an immediate stress-busting fix, the best way to clear your head is with relaxation breathing. If your day is extra stressful, you can use this breathing exercise each time you do some working on the ball to get out of your head and into the moment.

Start by sitting up straight with your feet firmly planted on the ground. Inhale slowly to a count of eight and exhale slowly to a count of eight. Expand your stomach on the inhalation and shrink your stomach on the exhalation. Focus on the physical sensations you experience during each breath. Repeat for one or two minutes. You can do this breathing exercise while you work at your computer,

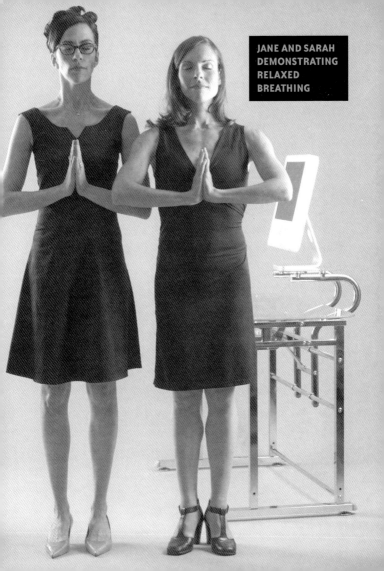

JANE AND SARAH
DEMONSTRATING
RELAXED
BREATHING

during a stressful meeting or phone call, or during a bathroom break to bring yourself back to a calm place. No one even has to know you're doing it.

General Tips

- Always be aware of your good posture and the position of your spine. Unless stated otherwise, your back should be in neutral. Refer back to page 16 and complete the posture test or follow the instructions on page 40 for a reminder of what good posture feels like.

- Think about what you're doing in each of the exercises. Move with control and be smooth, like butter. No jerkiness.

- Zero in on the body part you're trying to work in each exercise. Make sure that's where you're feeling the most effort. Visualization of the actual body part is very important.

- Breathe. Don't hold your breath; exhale on the hard part of the exercise and inhale on the easy part.

- Be hard on yourself. You can go through the motions and complete the exercises, or you can challenge yourself by creating extra resistance, making the air feel heavier (like moving through water), or making yourself feel heavier.

- Don't take yourself too seriously. Life can get dreary fast if you let it.

Getting Ball-Ready

The way you start your day will have a profound impact on the way the rest of your day goes. Before you get to your ball, you need to think about a routine that will ensure that you make healthy choices for your mind and body. Without a routine, it can be easy to let small things get you off track. Here are some tips to get you off on the right foot every day:

- Put your keys in the same place every night so you don't panic when you can't find them.
- Get your clothes and anything you need to take to work ready the night before.
- Create a peaceful environment to ease yourself into waking up. No news—just soft music.
- Wake up a few minutes before anyone else in the house and do two minutes of relaxation breathing.
- Drink a glass of water as soon as you get up.

- Get up early enough to eat a healthy, balanced breakfast that includes a complex carbohydrate and protein. Examples: yogurt, fruit, and granola; hard-boiled egg and whole-grain toast; cottage cheese, fruit, and a handful of almonds; slow-cooked oatmeal with sunflower seeds and frozen berries; yogurt and fruit smoothie.

- Decide how you're going to deal with a potentially stressful commute with something you look forward to, such as an audio book, the newspaper, or your favorite music.

Getting to *the Ball*

On your way to the office you can choose to think about all the work waiting for you on your desk or you can choose to focus on something you have more control over in the moment. You can focus on the commuters or drivers that are annoying you or you can visualize a successful day or productive meeting you've been preparing for. It's up to you. Wherever your thoughts go, your energy and vitality will follow.

The *Working on the Ball* way is there for you to choose:

- Reshape your perception of your surroundings and your surroundings will change with your new perceptions.

- Observe the hustle and bustle around without judgment instead of turning into one of the commuting zombies.

- You may learn something that changes your way of thinking or meet someone who influences you profoundly.

- Tell yourself that you love the time to yourself while you're headed off to work.

- Think of one thing you're excited about that's waiting for you at work.

Having a Ball on the Job

Start the

DAY off

on the

right side

of the

BALL.

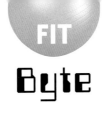

FIT

Byte

Go Easy **on the Java!**

Can't seem to start your day without your favorite brew? No big deal. A cup of great coffee actually improves alertness and energy. Who doesn't crave that? However, the fourth and fifth mugful can unleash a slew of unattractive qualities: jitters, restlessness, anxiety, insomnia, high blood pressure, and finally gut rot. If you don't want to seem like you're coming off a bad trip, stay under three cups a day.

The *Big Sit*

Seem as if it's too early in the day to tackle that mound of work piled high on your desk? How about an exercise program that begins with *sitting*? Before you go head to head with your professional obligations, take a moment and get centered for your busy day ahead. Have a seat on your ball and "PAC" it all in. PAC stands for:

Puppet: Stretch your head and torso upward, as if someone is hoisting you up with a string through the top of your head.

Anti-pee: Engage your anti-pee muscles—in other words, the muscles that stop you from peeing. (This exercise is also known as Kegels.)

Corset: Pretend someone just zipped a sexy corset around your waist, and suck your stomach into your back.

Now try breathing deeply, pulling the air down into the bottom of your stomach. There's a lot to pay attention to, but this will become habit over time. Imprint the way your body feels when you "PAC" it all in. This simple exercise is the foundation for the rest of the exercises in the book and for good posture while sitting on your ball.

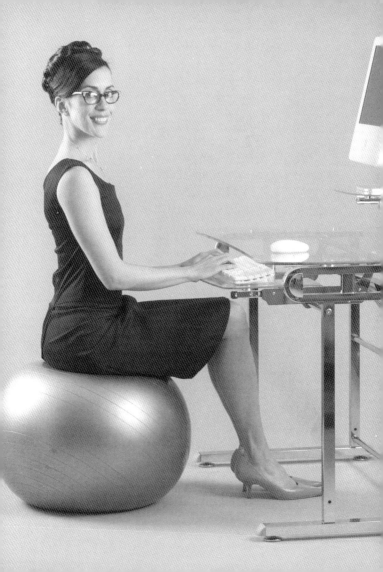

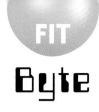

Byte

Eat Breakfast *to Lose Weight*

Had your oatmeal yet? An egg? Some toast? Anything?
You may think you're saving calories or outfoxing your
appetite, but research shows that people who skip
breakfast are more likely to overeat later in the day.
Eating protein and complex carbohydrates in the morning helps keep blood sugar and insulin levels regu-
lated. That way you won't be eating stale baked goods
at morning meetings or scraping change from the bottom of your purse at eleven A.M. in preparation for a
covert excursion to the vending machine.

The *Heel Digger*

S taff meeting starts in five minutes. Anxiety plus bad coffee and stale Danishes await your arrival. *Danishes? Hmmm . . .* Still, you're not ready to face the head honchos. Be a heel-digger and repeat, "I will not go to the meeting (yet). I will tone my butt instead!" To resist the temptation to enter the boardroom early and eat yesterday's day-olds, sit tall on your ball and PAC it in. Dig those heels into the ground. Then squeezing your butt, slightly lift off the ball. Slowly squeeze, relax . . . squeeze, relax . . . squeeze, relax. Repeat fifteen to twenty times. Dutiful dawdle completed, head down the hall. We're betting that with this prep you won't even want the strudel.

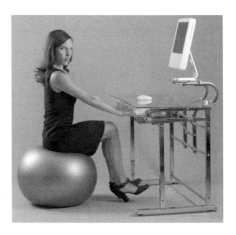

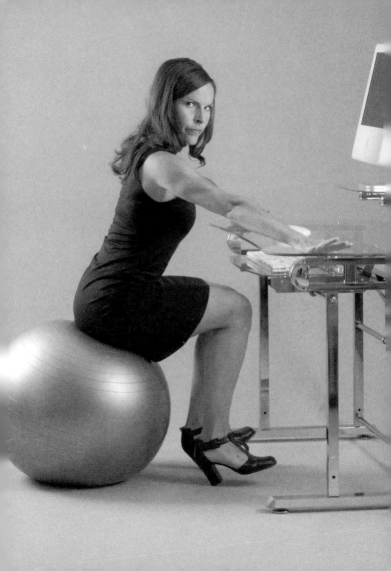

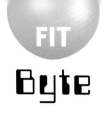

FIT

Byte

Focus on **Your Successes**

Events may sometimes beat you down, but don't do it to yourself! The happiest people spend the least amount of time thinking about what's wrong with themselves. Instead they focus on the positives in their lives, the good things that originate from their best qualities. To reinforce this, they concentrate on and emphasize what they do best. Just like anything that takes practice to perfect, getting "good" at exercise can take time. Challenges at the beginning will disappear with regular training. Keep a list of your five to ten best qualities or talents in your Palm Pilot or wallet, things that you feel you're really good at. Consult this list every time you feel blue.

Duck and *Cover*

*U*h-oh. The boss is stalking raptorlike down the hall, looking for you. Alert! Alert! Is it about the assignment you were supposed to hand in this morning? Or maybe you should've been at the meeting after all? Time to duck and cover! Make sure you're squarely seated on the ball, then PAC it in. Keeping your back neutral, bring your chest down toward your knees. Reemerge when the coast is clear, bringing your back up. Feel a nice lengthening through your spine and out through the top of your head.

For a more advanced movement, reach your arms straight up and keep them at your ears as you bend over. Repeat fifteen to twenty times.

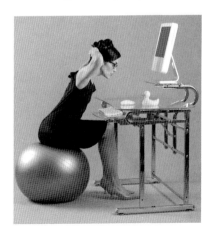

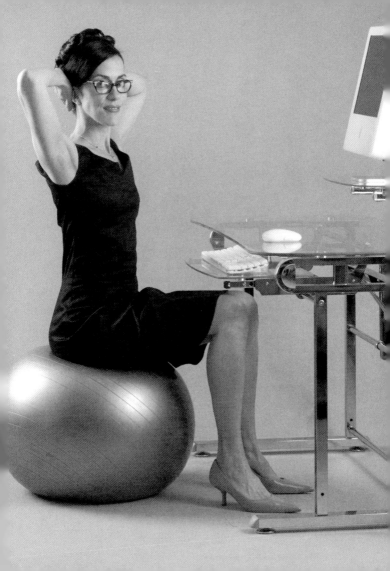

Midmorning
energy

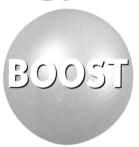

BOOST

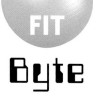

Byte

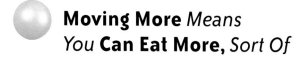

Moving More *Means You* **Can Eat More,** *Sort Of*

Use this quick formula to figure out the bare minimum of daily calories you need to maintain your weight: Divide your weight in pounds by 2.2, and multiply that number by 21.6. Next, if you are sedentary multiply this number by 1.25; if you are mildly active multiply it by 1.4; and if you are moderately active multiply it by 1.55. For example, a 145-pound woman who is mildly active should eat 1,993 calories a day to maintain her weight. Starving your body to become an instant size 6 is the fastest way to fail. You'll slow down your metabolism, get irritable, and turn yourself into a calorie-deprived psycho! Portion control, healthy eating, and increased exercise is a surefire path to long-term weight loss.

The *Hula*

I s your mind trailing off again to faraway places, beaches, grass skirts, and swimsuits? *Swimsuits*! Instead of getting panicky and scanning the horizon for a big palm frond to hide behind, better to get your bod bathing suit–ready! PAC it in. Squeeze those abs and move the hips side to side. The ball will move slightly with you. Resist moving quickly, and imagine that your waist is shrinking as you do ten to fifteen full hulas. Feel the breeze from the ocean, smell the salt and suntan lotion. Ah, so much fun to get "lei'd" at the office.

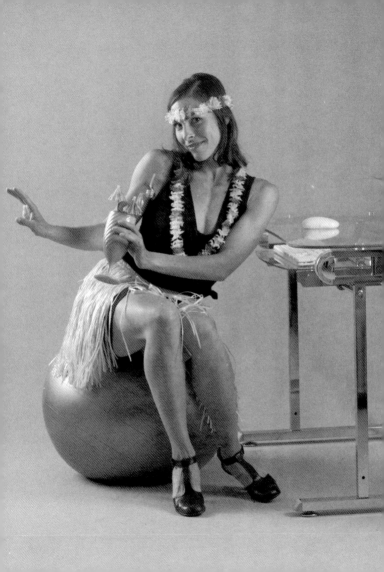

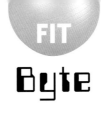

FIT
Byte

Start Your Day **with a Healthy** *Choice!*

Did you know that all your choices throughout the day or week become a part of a larger behavior chain? If you make a healthy lifestyle choice in the morning, you're less likely to indulge or skip exercise later in the day. If you break unhealthy links in these behavior chains, you might find yourself making healthier choices throughout your day or week. Avoid that cheesecake on Monday and you'll have a better chance of avoiding two pieces on Thursday.

The *Box*

Wow—look at you working away, making calls and being responsible. Clearly a little too square for the hula–mai tai thing. Okay, embrace your squareness. PAC it all in. Hips push forward to the right, back to the left, and to the front. Keep your movements small, precise, and controlled. Feel your entire core engage. Repeat for ten full boxes clockwise and ten counterclockwise.

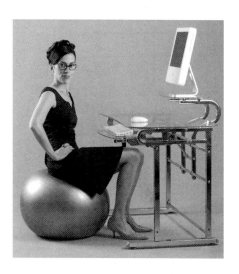

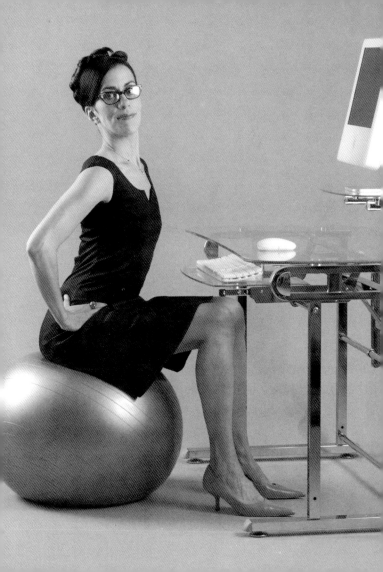

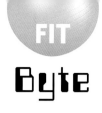

FIT

Byte

Seek Balance Between **Food Intake and Exercise!**

Seeking lifestyle balance has been a part of human existence for centuries. Did you know that the ancient Greeks were the first to write about fitness training? Hippocrates, who recommended that everyone walk after dinner, said that people are healthy when exercise and food are perfectly balanced. When the balance is off, people become ill. The guy in the toga may be long gone, but his ideas hold true.

Paperweight Relay

O n your desk, find the heaviest object that you can
hold in one hand. Lift it high over your head. Lean
forward on your ball, keeping your back neutral. Reach
out through the top of your head. PAC it in. Lower your
hands, then pass the object from one hand to the other
behind your back, keeping your arms straight. Then again
reach over your head. Make big circles over your head and
behind your back. Repeat ten times in each direction.

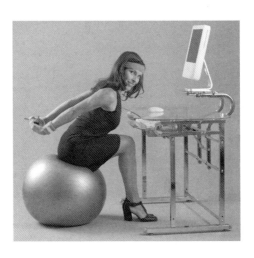

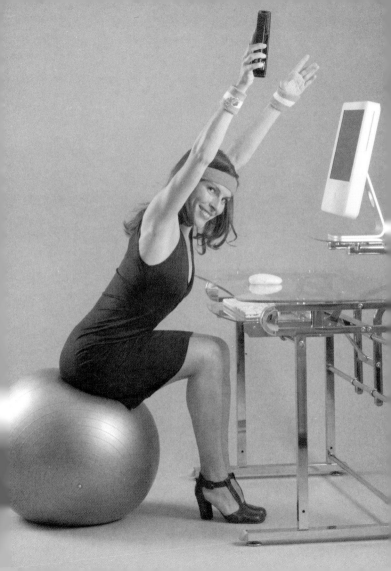

Take a **BREAK** from *sitting* and *shoes* *at* LUNCH.

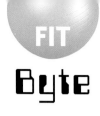

Byte

Shield Yourself *from Negativity*

Instead of letting people in your environment affect you negatively, reel your energy back and make your inner self inaccessible by creating an imaginary shield of protection around yourself. Imagine that you have cloaking armor circling you, making the negative vibes bounce right off and back at the source of the problem. Trust your gut about the people you need to protect yourself against. Remember, being known as the door mat in the office can get you in hot water. Sometimes you have to respectfully tell someone to shove it. Use the newfound strength from the physical work you're doing to further strengthen your shield. Think of the song "U Can't Touch This," and put a Buddha smile on your face.

The *Creep*

O h, man, here he comes! The office creep. Stalking you like prey, he wants to have lunch with you . . . again! Or maybe he wants to borrow your stapler, a pen, your mouse, your *whatever*. Time to hide! PAC it in. Slowly, stealthily, steadily creep under your desk. Take four steps forward. As you step, allow your spine to make contact with the ball one vertebra at a time. Just as slowly, walk back out and repeat ten times, until he's gone for sure.

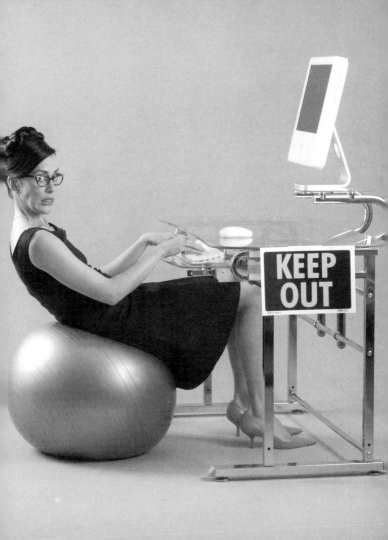

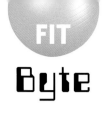

FIT

Byte

*You're Going on a **Trip— Pack Lightly!***

Wherever you go, your baggage goes with you. No amount of vacationing or escaping will get you away from your concerns, anxieties, or worries. Only constructive repatterning of your day-to-day living and thinking will lighten the load you carry wherever you go. Giving yourself time to clear your head will help you prioritize the backlog of thoughts that are crowding your mind. Getting into the moment by experiencing your physical self is the ticket that will take you on this journey.

Airplane

Want to fly away from all your worries? Maybe play hooky this afternoon? Not going to happen. So instead, let's pretend. PAC it in. Raise your arms straight out to the side at shoulder height and pull them back, squeezing your shoulder blades together. Hold your arms there. Hinge forward, sticking your butt back, with your palms toward the floor, and reach your tailbone up slightly toward the office ceiling. Keep your back neutral and shoulders down, and squeeze your upper back muscles together. Take five to ten long relaxation breaths and feel your worries take off.

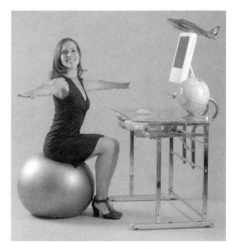

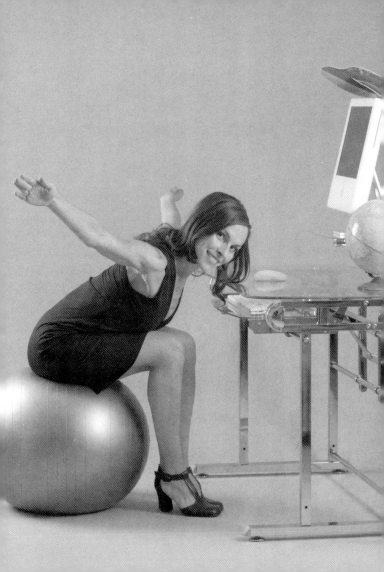

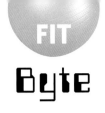

FIT
Byte

Balance *Your Body;*
Your Mind **Will Follow**

Before you can see the world around you clearly,
you need to create equilibrium in your very core.
Otherwise, it's like the world around you is an unpre-
dictable weather system and you're a dinghy rocking
back and forth on an ocean that is all too frequently
stormy. You need to get your body firmly grounded,
balanced, off the boat, and onto solid ground. Don't
let life's craziness turn you into a basket case.

Make Like a *Mountain*

Terra firma is calling your name. Ground yourself and imagine you're as solid as a mountain. Sit up tall and PAC it in. Extend your arms straight out in front of you just above shoulder height, palms down. Lift your butt off the ball and push your tailbone back, as if you were about to pee at a public toilet and can't touch the seat. Hover there and make sure you're balanced. Once you feel like you've achieved stability, hold for as long as you can stay balanced. Tip: Don't sit back down until you're sure the ball is under you. You should feel this working your thighs.

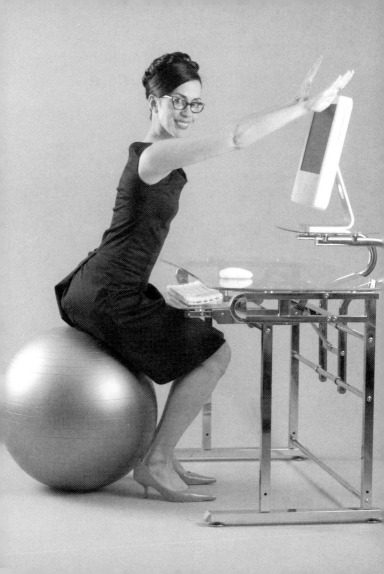

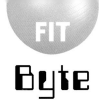

FIT

Byte

"I Rock My World, **I Rock My World,** *I Rock My World"*

Create mantras for yourself to avoid getting caught up in any surrounding negativity. It's so draining on your mind, body, and soul. Choose to resist societal pressures to judge yourself and others based on physical appearance. Respect yourself and others for strength of character. Give others credit for their accomplishments—and give yourself credit, too.

Rockin' Butt

Unless you can find a pair of those built-in-butt jeans, we'd better bring your derriere to the perkier side of things. Stand with your back toward the wall. Place the ball in the middle of your back, between you and the wall. Walk your feet out about four to six steps, so that you feel more of your body weight in your heels. Your legs should be hip width apart, with your knees and toes pointing in the same direction. PAC it in and keep your chest open as you bend your knees and send your butt toward the wall. You should feel like you're going to sit on the toilet. At the bottom of the movement, stop before your knees reach a ninety-degree angle. Then press your heels into the ground, squeeze your butt, and come back to standing. Keep going slowly down and up for twelve to fifteen smooth repetitions, exhaling on the way up and inhaling on the way down.

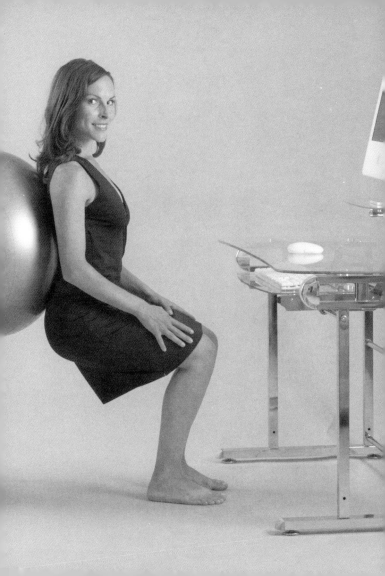

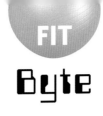

FIT

Byte

The Facts *Behind the Myths*

- *No pain no gain.* Yes. Exercise should be challenging and burning is allowed. However, there is such a thing as bad pain while you work out. Nothing should be sharp or sudden or alarming.

- *Resistance training will make you gain muscle bulk.* Yes. If you're taking steroids and lifting more than your body weight. Not if you're working on the ball. Our exercises will help you build long and lean muscles.

- *Exercising on an empty stomach will burn more fat stores.* Yes. But you're like an engine without fuel. You won't have the energy to push yourself. As a result, you will burn fewer calories overall. Weight loss is about calories consumed versus calories burned.

- *Eating before bed makes you fat.* Yes, if you've already consumed all the calories you need for the day. There's nothing magic about the midnight hour. If you need to snack before bed, eat a lighter dinner or choose a healthier low-calorie snack.

Upper-Back *Clap*

Working on the ball is a crazy thing. Nobody is going to applaud your work before you give yourself the kudos you deserve! Sit up tall, PAC it in, and slowly clap those hands behind your back at least twenty times, squeezing your shoulder blades together . . . really, you are worth it! Repeat two or three times, until the space between your shoulder blades burns.

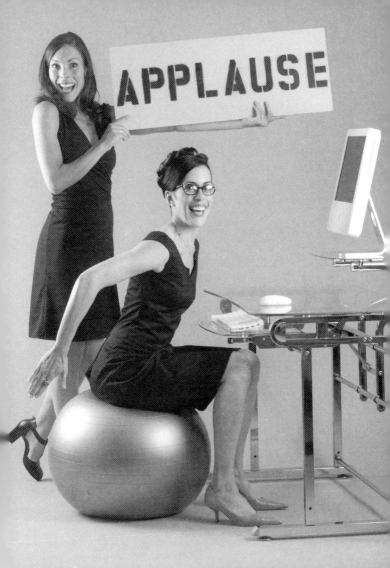

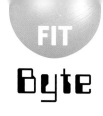

FIT

Byte

Your **Body Is Talking.** *Listen Hard!*

Repeatedly gaining and losing weight (yo-yoing) can give you the false impression that you have control over your body, but it may weaken your immune system in the long term. You'd better make peace with your body and accept its natural size and shape. Celebrate what your body can do for you and fuel it with a variety of healthful foods, enough rest, exercise, and, most important, respect. Taking care of your body's basic needs will help you gradually shed excess pounds.

Crunch Abs, Not Fritos

That bag of chips may be calling your name, but listen to your belly instead. Wouldn't you rather feel those muscles getting tighter, instead of your jeans? Begin by sitting tall. PAC it in and slowly walk your feet out ahead of you, letting your body slide along the ball, hang on to your desk for balance, until your lower back is pressing into the ball. Keep your shoulder blades off the ball, though. Put your hands across your chest if you're just starting out, or behind your head if you regularly do crunches. Squeeze your belly button down toward the ball as you exhale and slowly crunch up, keeping your chin off your chest. Bring your upper body up about six inches, then slowly down. Keep crunching for at least twenty repetitions and then slowly roll back up to sitting.

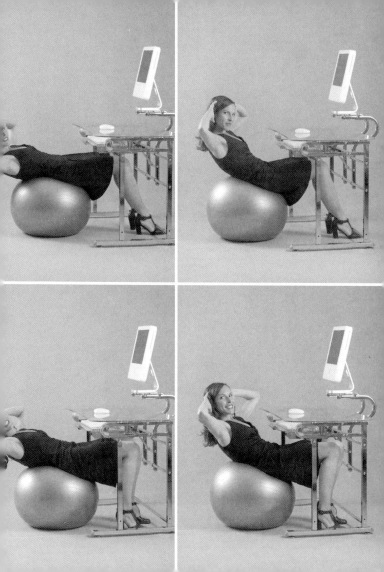

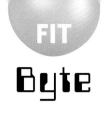

FIT

Byte

Indulge **Within Reason** *or* *Accept* **the Consequences!**

You've heard it said that a moment on your lips is instantly transported to your hips. It takes 3,500 calories of excess intake to create one pound of fat on the body. A jump on the scale after a night of overindulgence may be due to water retention and food bulk. However, a few days of pigging out and not working out is all it takes to hit that 3,500-calorie mark, thus making you question why your jeans are suddenly so snug. Nope, they haven't just been washed. Who needs a scale when you have the very telling and unforgiving denim gods?

Saddle Up
(and Ride Off into the Sunset)

How great would it be to straddle a horse and ride off into the sunset? Well you've got a ball and an imagination, so saddle up. Grab your desk firmly and straddle the ball, then lift your feet off the ground. Squeeze with your inner thighs and slowly let your body pull away from your desk as your arms straighten. Then engage those abs and slowly pull yourself back toward your desk. Keep squeezing the ball tight with your legs and continue for fifteen to twenty smooth and controlled repetitions.

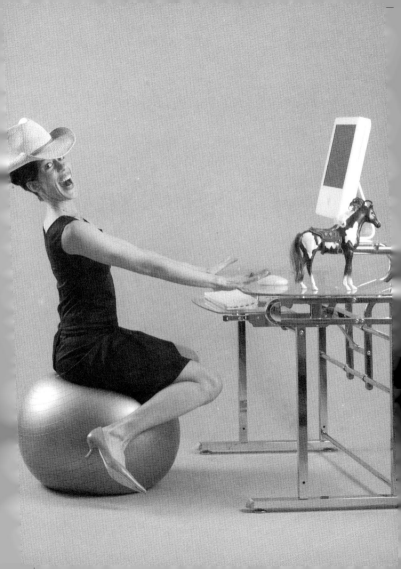

Settle
back
onto the
BALL
after
lunch!

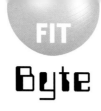

FIT

Byte

Find a **Reason to Move!**

Don't get discouraged if you can't make it to the gym—take mini-breaks from your desk as often as possible throughout the day to get your cardio in. If your coworkers ask where you're going again just tell them it's a stomach thing and take a power walk the long way around the office. Those little fast walks could translate into a twenty-minute workout by the end of the day. And we know it all adds up! Your colleagues will wonder why you're so sweaty whenever you come back from the loo, but they won't ask.

Ballsy *Bounce*

Okay. Lunch is over, digestion is occurring, and that tryptophan from your turkey sandwich is hitting your bloodstream. Sleep is very tempting, but it's wrong at the office. You need a pick-me-up. PAC it in and for thirty seconds bounce like there's no tomorrow. Come on, have a ball . . . faster, higher—nobody's looking!

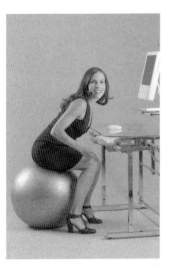 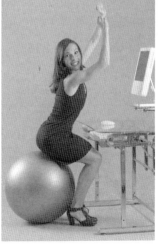

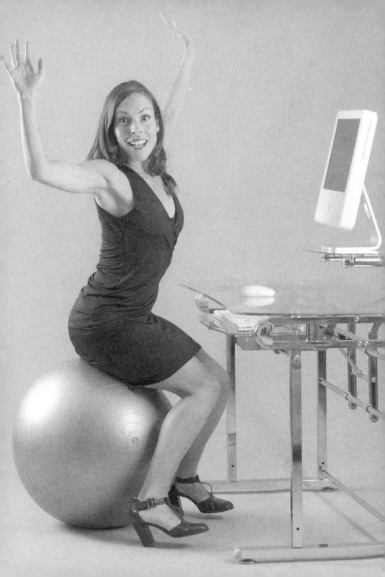

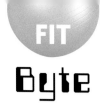

FIT
Byte

Don't Use Eating *as a Way to Pass Time!*

Some days are long and hard and there seems to be no escape from the overhead fluorescent lights. Instead of digging mindlessly into an unhealthy snack to feed your emotions and stave off boredom, get moving, call a friend, take deep breaths, or, better yet, close your eyes and take a five-minute stretching or meditation session. Your body and brain will thank you for the break and rejuvenation.

Tick *Tock*

O h, when will this day end? The clock seems to be moving in slow motion, and the buzz of your computer is lulling you into a comatose state. Time for a pick-me-up: take time into your own hands . . . and feet. Make like the hands of the clock and tick-tock your way around the ball. Start by sitting and PAC it in. Step one foot out to the side, rotating your body to face the direction of your foot, and bring the other foot in to meet it. Continue stepping out and bringing the other leg and foot in until you have made a complete rotation around the ball. Ensure all your movements are slow and controlled. The ball may turn with you. Repeat in the other direction for a complete circle.

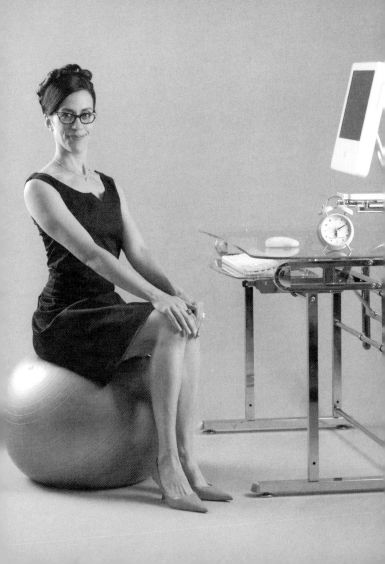

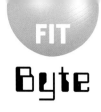

FIT

Byte

More Moving,
Fewer Ugly Veins!

Sitting in a stationary position for extended periods
can cause blood to pool in your legs, turning your poor
lower vascular system into a long tangle of overinflated
balloons. This results in stiffness and ... yikes! ... blood
clots. Performing small leg and ankle movements at least
once an hour will keep the blood flowing and diminish
the stress on your veins.

Best Foot *Forward*

After hours at your desk, trying to finish the last-minute details of your presentation, it's time to shine at the boardroom meeting. This is definitely not the moment for nerves and wobbly knees. Pep up and put your best foot forward before you waltz into that room. Start sitting and PAC it in, with your hands resting on the desk (for beginners), on your hips (for the more experienced), or with your palms squeezed behind your back (for the advanced). Extend one leg out in front of you. Do ten little circles in midair, then reverse the direction of the circle. Repeat with the other leg, because it, too, must be at its best. This may sound goofy, but you'll find that the exercise builds grace and helps develop heat and power in your body.

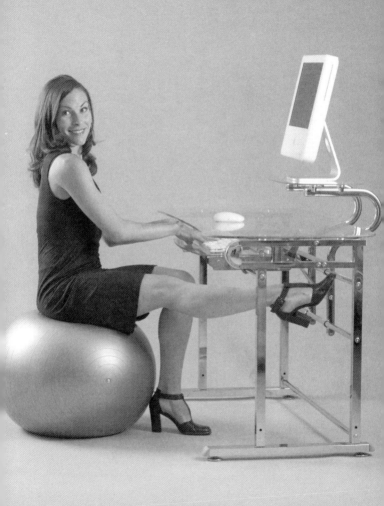

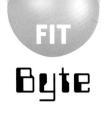

FIT

Byte

Create a **Tranquil Space at Your Desk,** *Ommmm*

So why not meditate for a few moments at the office? Your coworkers already think you're bonkers. Who will have the last laugh when you are fit, healthy, and tranquil? Find a quiet moment and a space where you can try to block out outside noise. Even clearing off part of your desk off can reduce anxiety and help you find some inner peace. Take deep breaths in and out; focus on a word and repeat it over and over again. It can be any word that makes you feel safe, inspired, or calm. Try *peace . . . love . . . chocolate . . .*

Hoe Down

Wow—your project partner and you just got a nod from the bigwigs upstairs. Whew—time to celebrate . . . swing your partner round and round!

Now, on the ball, lift your knee up from the ground. Slowly move that knee up and down, squeezing your abs on each lift and keeping the rest of your body completely still. Think of a knee-slapping good time . . . work is such a ball! Yee-ha! Repeat fifteen times for each leg.

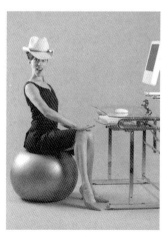
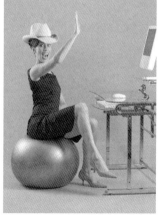

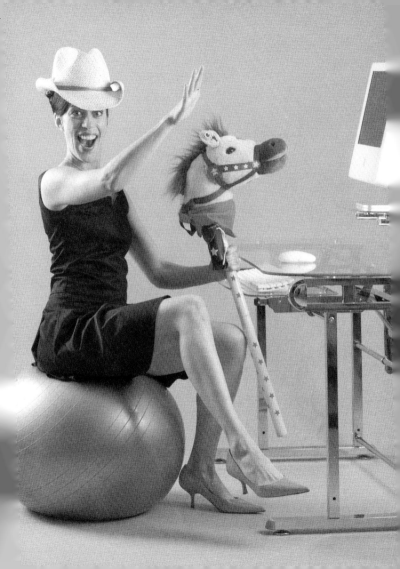

Mid*afternoon*

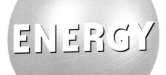

ENERGY

pick-me-*ups*

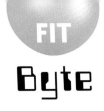

FIT

Byte

*Don't Let Stress Go **Too Far!***

Feeling a little stressed at work? Well, it's not such a bad thing now and then. A little stress can actually improve immune function, by upping antibodies when things are getting a bit tense. But chronic stress leads to a drop in those sickness-fighting antibodies, which weakens your resistance to infection. Feeling overwhelmed, run-down, and exhausted all the time? You must take steps to help your body, mind, and soul find some tranquillity—perhaps through meditation.

The *Buddha*

Can't make it to yoga today, again? Is it getting hard to concentrate as your mind takes you out of this work moment and on to what yummy naughty snack you could indulge in? Try some good old yoga instead. It's almost as tasty and equally satisfying. Sit up tall and PAC it in.

With your palms together in front of your chest, press your hands as hard as you can. Very slowly, lift your hands up overhead, still pressing your palms together, and slowly lower them, exhaling on the way down. Keep your chest open and proud. Repeat ten times with big Buddha breaths.

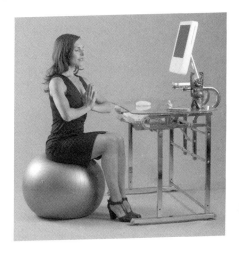

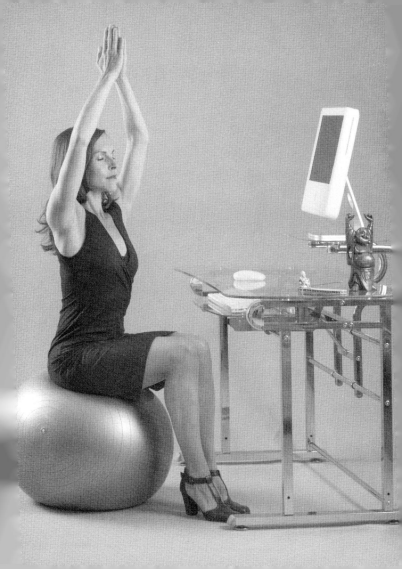

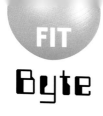

FIT

Byte

Take the **Stairs!**

Why on earth would you take the stairs when there's a good elevator opening its doors to you? For starters, you can burn about one calorie for every step you climb. On the way up, take them two steps at a time. Oh yeah—did we mention that you should take them twice just for fun?

Repeat: Take the stairs, will you?!

Robot *Twist*

Will this day ever end? Answer e-mails, staple proposals, do the crossword . . . automatic pilot has set in again. Some days you feel like a programmed robot. Turn off autopilot and remember . . . like you did last summer? That's right—let's twist!

Sit and PAC it in. Keep your hips facing forward and slowly twist your upper body side to side, feeling a tightening and lengthening through your waist. If you feel like a robot you are on the right track. Repeat ten times in each direction.

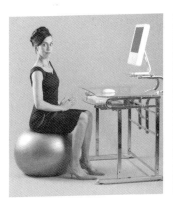
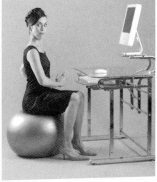

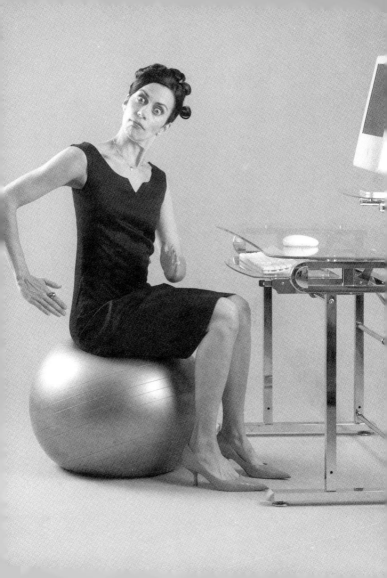

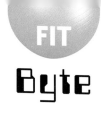

FIT

Byte

Stop. Think *Before You Eat!*

Love those office parties. *Happy birthday to you, happy birthday to you . . .* but not so happy that one piece of cake can easily cost you three hundred calories. Then there's the wine, one hundred calories per glass, and that damn chip bowl, six chips ringing in at seventy calories. To celebrate another office birthday for people you would never even buy a present for, you're putting away almost five hundred extra calories? Too much to sacrifice! Take an inventory of what you've eaten in your day before you reach for a special treat. . . . Stop, think, and then *maybe* eat.

The *Surrender*

Put your hands up over your head! You have surrendered to the idea of working hard, being a huge success, and looking totally sexy. Get your palms facing each other, keep your ball completely still, and don't let those shoulders sneak up toward your ears. Relax your shoulders while you reach your fingers up toward the ceiling. Slowly tip your body over to one side at the waist, keeping your arms right at the sides of your head. (Keep your movements small until you feel balanced and get the hang of it.) Come back to center and then tip over to the other side. Repeat on each side five to ten times.

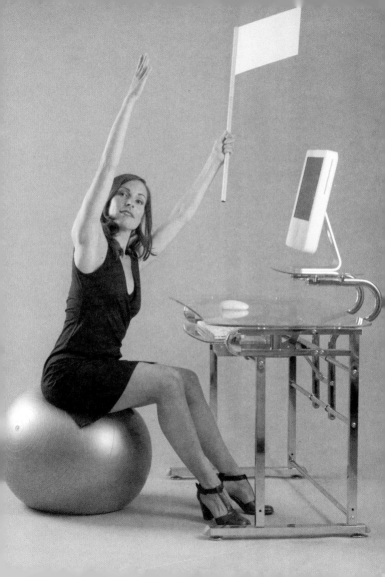

Finish the **DAY**

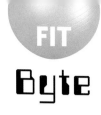

FIT

Byte

Stop **Procrastinating!**

Feel the need to be trendy? That's fine if it comes to being a fashionista, but in the fitness realm trends can be overrated. Many people spend more time reading fitness magazines than they do actually trying to get fit. Being too concerned with the perfect new butt or shoulder exercise might be a way to procrastinate. Getting fit is about moving more and watching what you eat. Just do it, for goodness' sake!

Closing the Deal

You did it—signed, sealed, and delivered! Rejoice, the deal is done!

This exercise is kind of like the heel-digger but more ballsy. Refer back to page 44 for a little refresher. Go higher and see what's over the top of that divider! Squeeze that butt as tight as you can. Maybe you feel a little anal-retentive, but your butt will thank you. Touch the ball with your fingers after each bounce just to make sure it's still there. Repeat fifteen to twenty times.

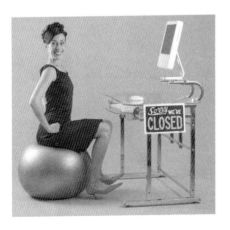

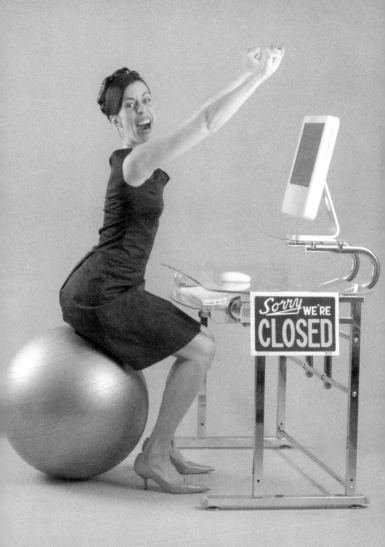

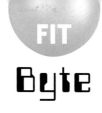

FIT

Byte

Trust the **Fitness Addicts!**

Most people start an exercise program to lose weight or tone up sagging muscles. But what they don't know is that consistent exercise elevates their mood due to the release of natural pain killers called endorphins. After three weeks of consistently using this book, you should start feeling the buzz endorphins provide. Just beware. As with any feel-good drug, you'll experience withdrawal if you stop exercising for more than a few days.

The *Scarecrow*

It's nearing the end of your day. Your makeup isn't perfect anymore, your hair not as coiffed as it once was, your skirt or pants wrinkled. You know you don't really look scary, but let's pretend for fun.

Sit tall and PAC it in. Lift your arms up level with your shoulders, your elbows bent at ninety degrees, and your palms facing forward. Tip your hands forward to shoulder height, then rotate them back behind your ears slightly. Move your arms slowly and imagine that someone is pushing against your palms to create extra resistance. Repeat fifteen to twenty times.

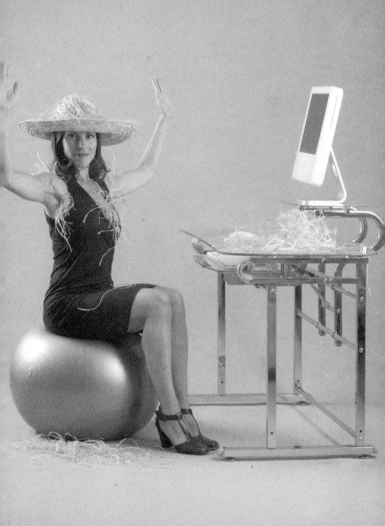

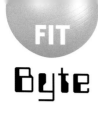

FIT

Byte

Save Gas! *Save Cash!*

Americans spend an average of 541 hours per year in cars. That's one and a half hours per day. That's almost 10 percent of our waking hours. No wonder people say they can't find time to exercise. Why not build exercise into your commute? If possible, run, walk, ride your bike, or even just park farther away from your workplace and walk partway. There are no excuses for not getting exercise, just poorly laid plans.

Had-Its

You've had it with the office politics. Why do they keep piling crappy assignments on your desk? Push it away and reap the benefits of a beautiful chest. With your hands wide on the edge of your desk and your feet off the ground, PAC it in and slowly lower your chest toward your desk. Keep your shoulders away from your ears and elbows pointing back and slightly down. Exhale on the way up. Repeat fifteen to twenty times times.

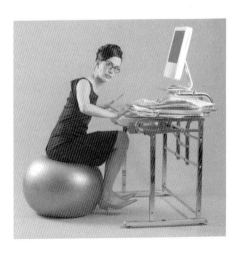

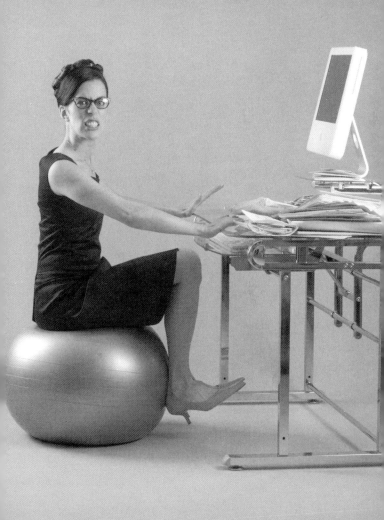

Working

LATE ...

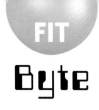

FIT

Byte

Choose *Your State of Mind!*

Stress is largely a function of how we perceive events or our environment. So maybe you have to work late tonight. You could get really frustrated or you could go with the flow and realize that no amount of anger will get you home faster. If you have to stay, then make the most of it. Don't make the situation more stressful by carrying tension in your body. Instead of trying to rush, which will get you out of your flow, take a couple of minutes to refocus and do some working on the ball.

Tabletop *Tango*

Ahhhh . . . finally everyone has gone home. Just you, your ball, and your butt. Before you strip out of your office attire and throw on those fab jeans, let's tighten that derriere! Start by sitting on the ball. PAC it in and slowly walk it out until your body is creating a flat tabletop position with your shoulders remaining on the ball. Slowly drop your bum toward the floor, then squeeze and slowly lift those hips toward the ceiling. Repeat twenty times. You should feel this exercise in your hamstrings, butt, and lower back.

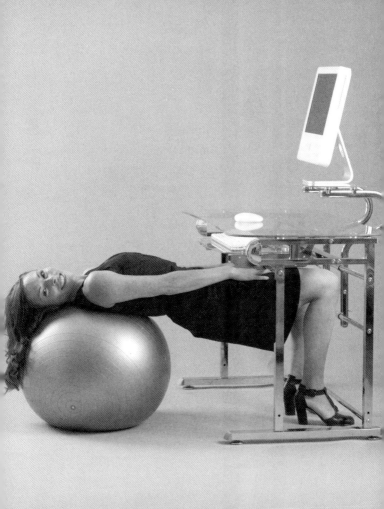

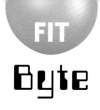

FIT

Byte

Embrace the Sexy You!

Now that you're alone, did you know that 14 percent of people have had sex at work? We're not saying go have a fling with someone in the broom closet, but these facts may help motivate you to get your work done ASAP!

You can burn lots of calories getting it on. Here are the figures:

Kissing	120–325 calories per hour, or 2–5 calories per minute
Taking care of yourself	100–150 calories per session
Average sex session	150–200 calories per session
Sex 3 times per week	23,000–31,000 calories per year (6.5–9 lbs. lost per year)

Pickups

Oops, you dropped something! Slowly reach down to your right side and pick up that pencil with your right hand, then reach to your left side and pick up that paper clip with your left hand. Keep your body facing straight forward and PAC it in. You don't have to actually touch the floor and you might not be able to. The ball will move under you slightly as you bend at each side. Try to keep your feet stationary and make sure you feel stable and balanced before going deeper in this movement. Do this ten times on each side. Your waist will thank you.

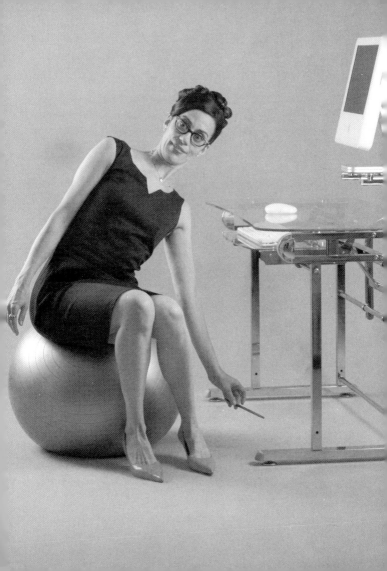

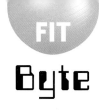

FIT

Byte

Always Take Care of
Yourself First

Occasionally feeling low, blah, wiped out, or down? Sometimes feel overwhelmed by the volume of work in front of you? Wish you could stay home in bed some days? Emotional fatigue might be the true cause. We have only so much to give. When you put out more than you're taking in, your tank goes empty. If you've been really low for a number of weeks, you might be depressed and need to talk to your doctor. You might have to find a way to say no more often and say yes to yourself. *Yes to a vacation, yes to a massage, yes to a hot bath, yes to a spa weekend, yes to a chocolate croissant . . .* Hey! Hey! Don't get too carried away.

A Different Sort of
Inflatable Date

Not so happy that you're still slogging away at work while everybody else is gone? Make some space for yourself and get to know your ball better. Lie on it, face-down, with your pelvis on the ball, up close and personal, nice and intimate. Try lifting your chest up to a neutral spine with your feet and knees on the ground. If you're a beginner, you should put your hands behind your head with your elbows out to the side. If you're more advanced, reach your arms straight out in front of you and keep your arms level with your ears. Hold this position for five to ten seconds and repeat five times. You should feel a muscle-fatigue sensation in your lower back, but anything sharp, pinching, or sudden means you need to take a break and work your way up to the full five- to ten-second hold.

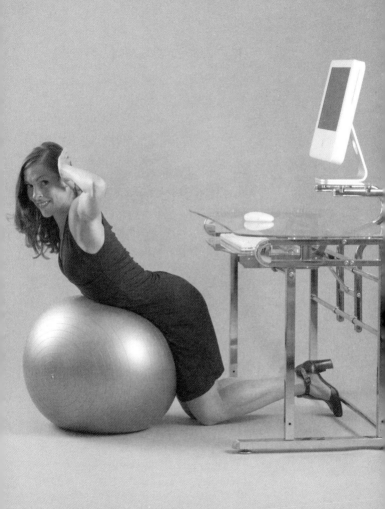

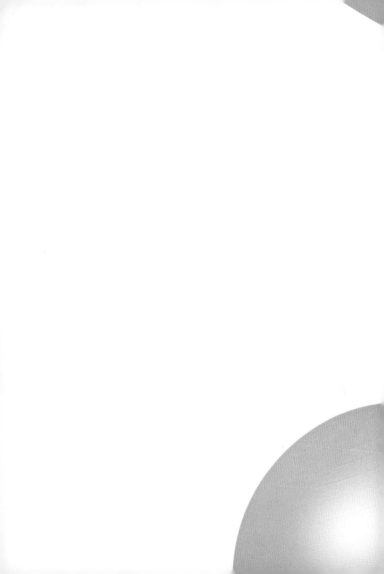

Dropping

the
Ball

Stretching at Your Desk

Did you know that the "high alert" feelings brought about by stress produce actual hormonal changes in your entire body? In prehistoric times, attacks from enemies or predators would have precipitated this state of readiness, preparing your body to take off or defend itself. Now, sitting inert at your desk, you feel the same degree of stress, but you're not running, you're not fighting, you're not moving your body. You're sedentary, bathing in hormonal changes without physical action. These hormones (cortisol mainly) make our bodies hang on to fat like it's going out of style and put it where we least want it, in our guts and around our organs. Having excess fat around our organs increases our risk for diabetes and heart disease. That's why activity is so important.

Stretching is an essential part of any fitness program and a definite must after strength training. It helps prevent injuries, increases range of motion in inflexible joints, and provides an opportunity to release negative energy. Stress and tension will find a place to rest in your body and give you ongoing grief for weeks or months unless you release them. Stretching provides a healthy alternative to what may be some destructive coping mechanisms. Sometimes the best thing to do is to release tension by giving your mind and body a chance to relax. Stretch and breathe. Take a moment at any point during the day to release tension in your neck, back, shoulders, or legs. Let the stress and tension out every time you exhale.

Body

Let It All *Hang Out*
(LOWER BACK)

While sitting on the ball, let your body fold forward over your thighs and release the tension in your neck, back, and arms. Let your head go loose like a big bowling ball hanging on a string. Nice deep breaths in, out, in, out . . . Hold for twenty to thirty seconds.

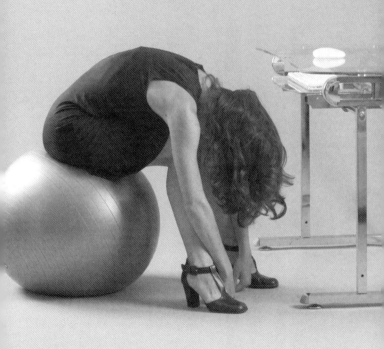

Body

Open *Your Heart,* and *Your Mind* Will Follow

(ENTIRE FRONT OF BODY)

Start in a sitting position on the ball and walk your feet out so that the ball is supporting your back and shoulders. Let your midback rest on the highest part of the ball. Release your head back and let your body feel long and heavy, as your arms open wide to the sides, opening your chest and rib cage. You should feel like a limp noodle. Stay limp and relaxed for twenty to thirty seconds.

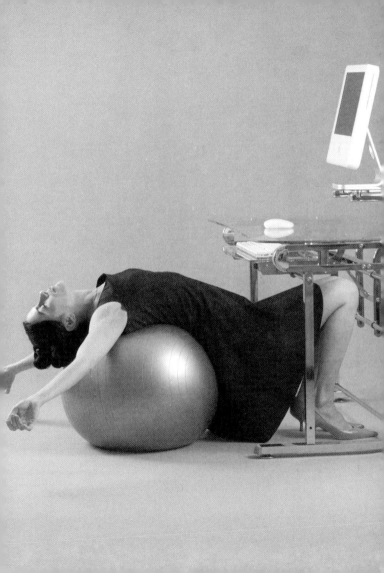

Body

Wrist *Twist*
(MUSCLES SURROUNDING WRIST)

S it up tall on the ball and take a moment to gently flex and bend each wrist. Then make slow circles outward and inward with both hands at the same time. It's a "joint" venture. Try to make the circles as big as possible. Crackling is normal as long as it doesn't hurt.

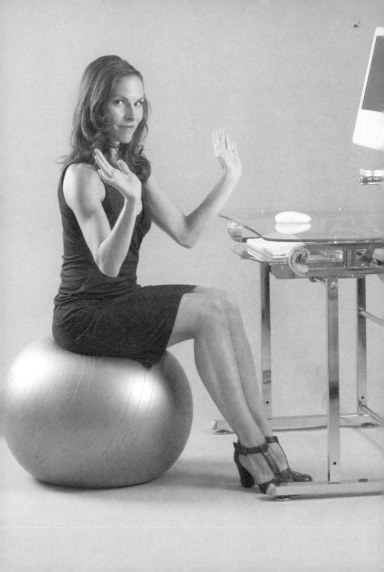

Body

Touch *the Ceiling*
(LATERAL UPPER-BODY MUSCLES)

From a sitting position, reach one arm up and over your head. Lean over slightly and rest your other hand on your stomach. Then reach your fingers toward the ceiling, lengthening the entire side of your upper body. Feel like you're pulling one side of your rib cage away from your hip bone. Keep your shoulder away from your ear. Hold for twenty to thirty seconds and remember to breathe. On exhalation, bring your body back to the center. Repeat on the other side.

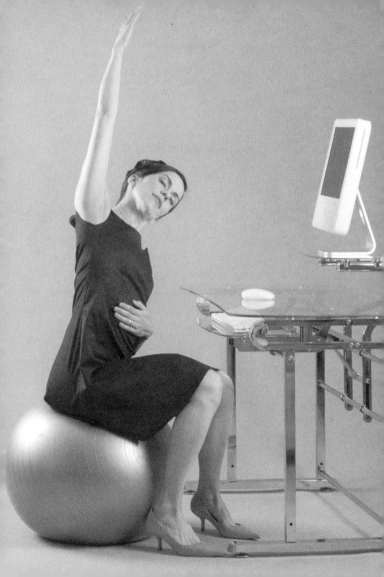

Body

Shoulder Blading
(UPPER BACK)

Sit up tall and clasp your hands in front of you. Rotate your palms until they are facing your computer monitor. Take a deep inhalation. As you exhale, press your palms toward the monitor and send your upper back toward the wall behind you. Round out your upper back and keep your shoulders down. Tuck your chin into your chest and hold for twenty to thirty seconds. Feel your shoulder blades pulling away from each other.

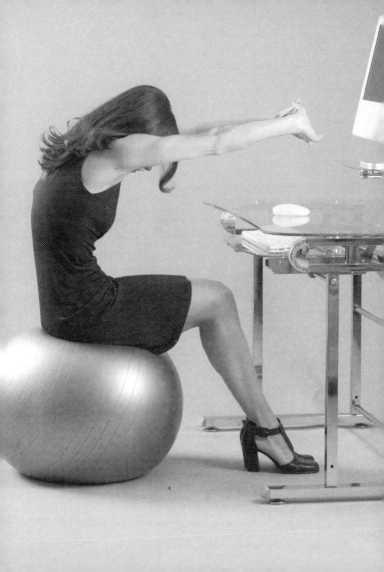

Body

Lat It *Up*
(BIG BACK MUSCLES—THE LATS)

Start in the same position as the previous exercise: clasp and rotate your hands. Inhale deeply and raise your hands over your head. Press your palms toward the ceiling as you pull your shoulders down. Make the distance between your hands and shoulders as long as possible. You should feel a stretch down your sides, right under your armpits. Try to keep your neck muscles relaxed as you extend your hands up and away. Hold for twenty to thirty seconds.

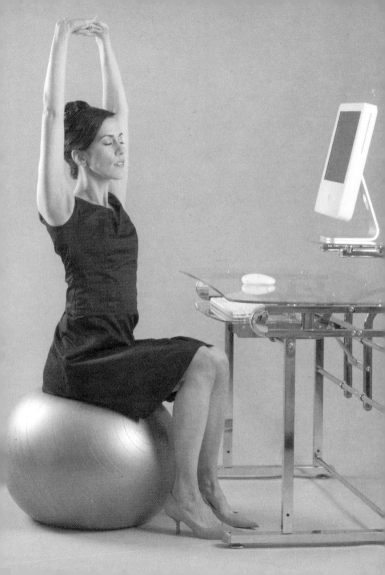

Body

Back *Scratch*
(TRICEPS, CHEST, FRONT OF SHOULDERS)

Reach over your head with one arm, drop your hand down toward your midback, and try to get your fingers between your shoulder blades. Take the other hand and press down on your raised elbow. You should feel a stretch down the back of your arm as you keep reaching your fingers down your back. Hold for twenty to thirty seconds. Repeat on the other side.

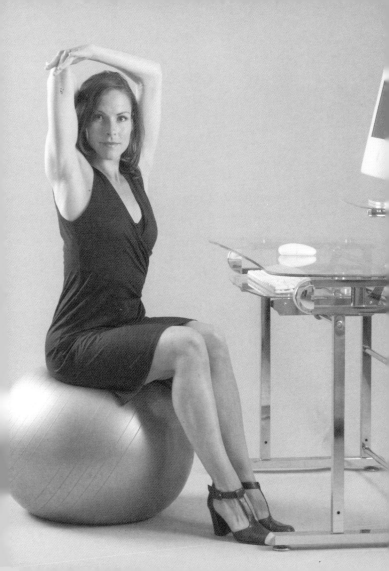

Body

Empty *the Woman's* Purse
(UPPER NECK AND SHOULDERS)

Some practitioners of ancient Chinese medicine refer to the upper neck muscles as the Woman's Purse, the place where we hold all of our emotional stress. Sit up tall, clasp your hands behind your back, and pull your hands down toward the floor. Gently, with an exhalation, let your head drop to one side. Hold for a few breaths, making your neck as long as possible, then let it circle in front of you, pulling your chin down to your chest. When you find an extra-tight spot, stay there for a few seconds and use your exhalation to release tension. Repeat the stretch, dropping your head to the opposite side.

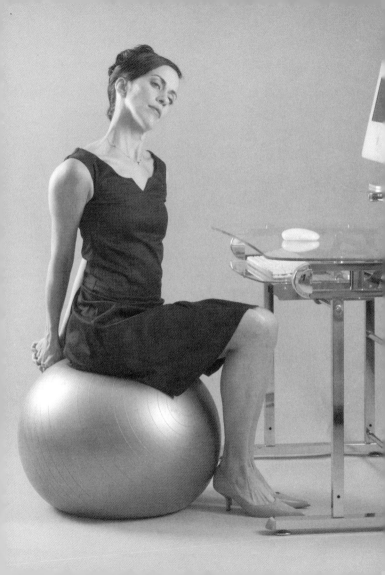

Body

Open Your *Insides*

(CHEST AND ABS)

Start by sitting tall and placing your hands on your kneecaps. Take a nice deep inhalation and lift your chest toward the ceiling, pull your ribs apart for twenty to thirty seconds, and allow your body to pull back slightly. Keep holding on to those knees for twenty to thirty seconds.

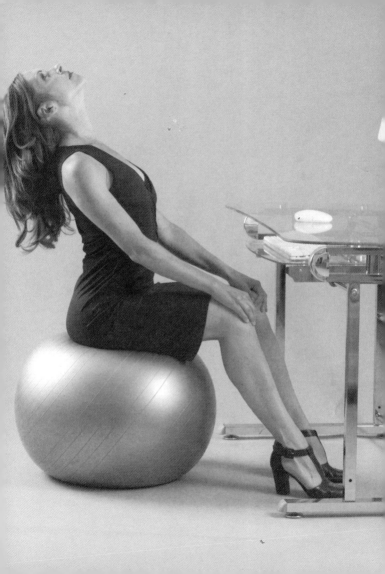

Body

We're on *Your Side*

(OBLIQUES—SIDE OF STOMACH)

Sitting up tall, raise one arm straight up toward the ceiling while the opposite arm is resting on the side of the ball. Take a deep breath in and on the exhalation reach the arm over your head toward the opposite wall. Hold for twenty to thirty seconds, then repeat on the other side.

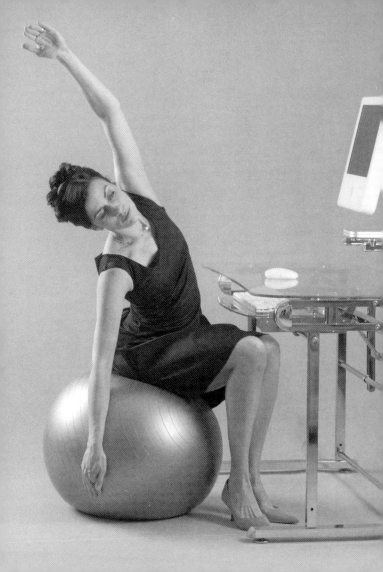

Body

Wring It Out
(BACK AND SIDES)

Start by sitting up tall, with your feet flat on the floor and your knees about hip width apart. Place your right palm on the outside of your left knee and your left hand behind you on the ball. As you take a deep breath, sit even taller. Apply gentle pressure to your knee with your right hand and rotate your upper body to the left side. Use your knee as resistance for your right hand. Keep your shoulders down and maintain good posture. Take five slow, deep breaths. Then return to the center and repeat on the other side.

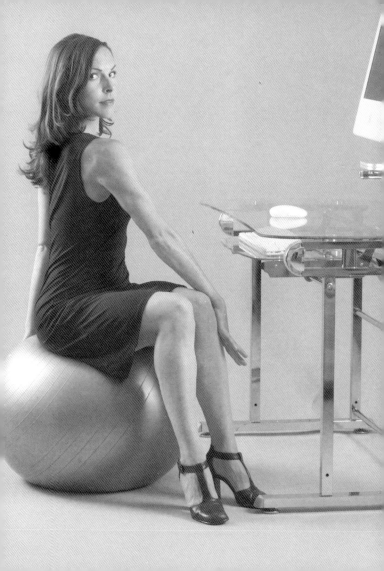

Body

Inner-Thigh Sigh

Start by sitting on ball. PAC it in and hold on to your desk. Position your legs on either side of the ball, knees facing the ceiling. (If you feel like a sumo wrestler, you're on the right track.) Gently, with control, straighten one leg as you allow the ball to move toward the bent leg. Hold through a few deep breaths, then take it to the other side.

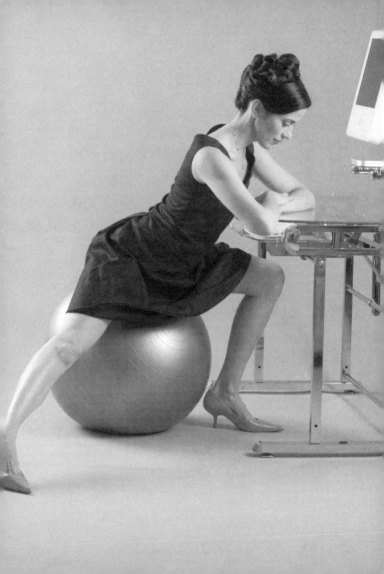

Body

No More *Tight* Asses
(BUTT)

S tart by sitting tall. Then reach down with your right hand to take hold of your right ankle. Hold on to your desk for stability with your opposite hand. Place your right foot on your left thigh just above the knee. As you inhale and exhale, gently roll the ball back about six inches and let your upper body fold forward. Try to keep that knee facing the wall, as opposed to the ceiling. Hold for twenty to thirty seconds. Don't forget the other side.

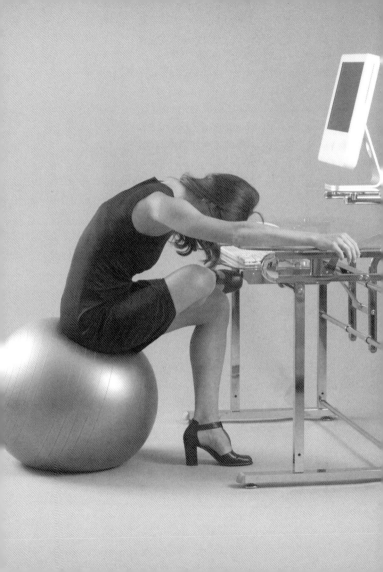

Body

Front-Thigh Sigh
(QUADS)

Sit up straight and reach down with your right hand to grab your right ankle. Hold on to your desk with your left hand for stability. Pull your ankle in toward your bum and press the inside of your knee into the ball. While breathing evenly keep reaching your knee toward the floor, pulling your ankle into your butt and your inner thigh into the ball. Hold for twenty to thirty seconds. Repeat on the other side.

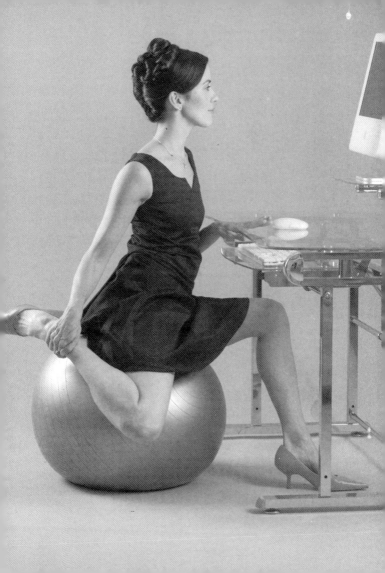

Body

Damn *Those Heels*

(CALVES)

PAC it in. Place two hands on your desk for support. Lift one leg up in front of you and flex your foot so that your toes are reaching back toward your nose. Hold for a few deep breaths and repeat on the other side.

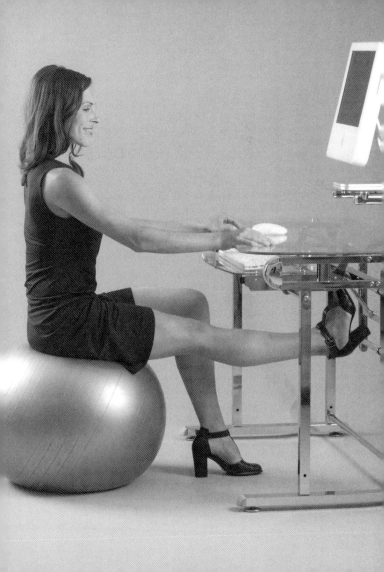

Body

Your *Aching* Feet

(FEET AND SHINS)

Slip off those shoes and PAC it in. Hold on tight to your desk. Point your right foot and place it on the floor beside you with your toe knuckles facing into the floor. Repeat with the left leg. Hold on to the desk with two hands. Gently rock the ball backward about four inches to feel a nice stretch through the top of the foot and shins.

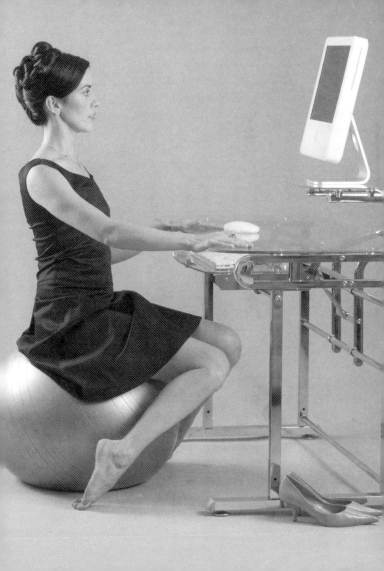

Leaving *the Ball*

Your workday is done, and now you get to welcome the commute home again. Here are some tips for making your commute a more relaxing event:

- Get a favorite CD and tune the outside noises out—unless, of course, you're driving in heavy traffic.

- Try recorded books. Not the motivational kind—the type that helps take your mind off achieving anything.

- Make a conscious choice about how you're going to let the hustle and bustle affect you. If you let it, it can make your life miserable.

- Smile at grumpy people. It's funny to watch their reactions. You might even get a smile back—or they might just think you're a little off your rocker.

- When you start to get tense because someone cut you off, think about PACing it in. Get into your body and out of your head. Relax your face, your jaw, in between your eyes, and breathe right down into the base of your stomach.

We thank you for being a part of *Working on the Ball* for the day. Remember all the work you've done. Do yourself proud and stay on track for tonight. Try to avoid those sugary or salty snacks that seduce you. Be nice to yourself. Take a bath. Have a little glass of wine or your favorite tea. Soak your feet and read your favorite novel or magazine. Think of what you did great today. There is no such thing as a wasted day.

Feeling More Ballsy . . .

After a month or two of consistently completing all the exercises in *Working on the Ball,* you can make things harder by:

- Adding a set to each exercise with a little twenty-second rest in between. After another month or two add one more set.

- Working your way up to being able to use the ball as a chair all day long.

- Using your mind to challenge yourself. Zero in on those muscles and create resistance in the air as you move.

- Picking up a copy of *Working on the Ball II* and getting started!

Acknowl*edgments*

Our thanks to our agent, Winifred Golden, to the talented Michael Alberstat for the smokin' photos, to Nora Underwood and Tershia d'Elgin for helping us edit, to Trisha Young for makeup, to Johanne Williams for hair, to Sabina for her creative input, to Sandra Ricciuto at Level V, and to Erin Friedrich at Andrews McMeel.

A special thanks from Jane to my husband, Rob, and my beautiful girls, Chase and Cheyne. You give me direction and purpose. A big thanks to my clients, who inspire me to be great.

A special thanks from Sarah to Dena Zimbel and my son, Logan.

the *Authors*

Jane **Clapp**

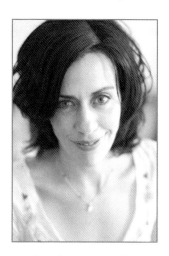

Jane has spent thirteen years as a fitness professional refining her knowledge and skills while working with hundreds of clients and class participants. Her potent brew of training alchemy blends functional training, weight management, lifestyle consulting, and stress management to proven effect. Jane is the founder of Urbanfitt, a personal and corporate fitness services company that caters to a discerning clientele. Her client roster includes high-profile urban professionals and celebrities such as Richard Dreyfuss and Daniel Richler. She also delivers fitness leadership training for corporate wellness facilities.

Jane earned her bachelor of commerce degree specializing in human resource management and later completed an intensive negotiation and mediations skill program. Her experience working for large corporations in change management, employee wellness, and training resulted in the creation of a distinctive fitness approach that addresses the specific challenges a desk worker faces.

Jane is a certified personal trainer with CPTN, a weight management and lifestyle consultant with ACE, a pre- and postnatal specialist with Can Fit Pro, and a Nike fusion specialist.

Jane has been a guest on radio and talk shows and hosted Toronto Film Festival events. She is a freelance fitness writer and her interviews have appeared in several national newspapers and magazines.

Sarah **Robichaud**

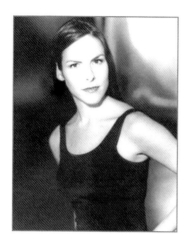

Sarah is a classically trained dancer who has performed extensively throughout Canada and the U.K. and in Moscow, where she spent two years at the Bolshoi Ballet School. Her drive and passion for an optimum mind-body connection in her dance career led her away from the dance studio and into the gym. There, Sarah fused her dance training with functional resistance exercises to help her clients and dance students attain long, lean muscle tone and improved posture. To help others achieve strong cores and lengthened muscles, she developed a ballet boot camp class that combines ballet and contemporary gym exercises for nondancers.

Sarah is a certified personal trainer with a client roster that spans every age and ability. She has a found a niche training established actors boot-camp style to get them buff and camera-ready. Most recently, she has helped Cary Shields, Broadway star of *Rent,* to look and feel fit enough to breeze through his grueling schedule of eight shows a week.

Sarah has choreographed and performed for many large productions both in the theater and on TV, and continues to actively pursue her career in the arts. Her best gig so far is having the joy of raising her son, Logan.